NOCTURNAL LEG CRAMPS
And Other Leg Muscle Pains
Causes, Risk Factors, Treatment, and Prevention

Pierre Mouchette

Life-Health Media USA
Enviro | Life Knowledge Publications

ISBN 9798853652439 (Paperback Edition)

Independently Published
Enviro | Life Knowledge Publications

First Edition: July 2023
Life-Health Media USA
https://www.enviro-life-media.com/

Disclaimer

Life-Health Media USA writers provide applicable content and break down complex topics, making them easier to understand. The information given may not apply to your situation, and the products or services recommended may not be a good fit for your application. While Life-Health Media USA strives to provide accurate, up-to-date content, we cannot guarantee the accuracy and completeness of the information supplied.

The author and publisher of this publication are not acting as licensed professionals in the presentation of this writing. Information, statements, and data provided are for educational purposes and do not replace a one-on-one relationship with any licensed professional required by Federal, State, County, or Local Government. The reader is solely responsible for the use of all content and holds Life-Health Media USA, Enviro | Life Knowledge Publications, and its members harmless in any event or claim, demand, or damage, including reasonable attorneys' fees, asserted by any third party, or arising out of your use of or conduct on publications and products.

INFORMATION - USE and DISCLAIMER

This generalized information is a limited diagnosis, treatment, and medication summary. It is not intended to be comprehensive and should only be used to help the user understand and consider potential diagnostic and treatment options. All information concerning conditions, treatments, medications, side effects, and risks that may apply may not be included. Information given is not intended to be medical advice or a substitute for a health care provider's diagnosis or treatment established on the provider's examination and assessment of the individual's specific and unique conditions. Patients must communicate with a health care provider for comprehensive information concerning health, medical questions, and treatment options, including risks or benefits regarding the use of medications. This information does not endorse any treatments or drugs as safe, effective, or approved for treating a specific patient.

Table of Contents

CHAPTER 1
NOCTURNAL LEG CRAMPS

Nocturnal leg cramps are a tight, knotted feeling in your legs at night. The pain can last for several seconds to several minutes, and the muscle can be sore for several days if the cramp is severe. Nevertheless, nocturnal leg cramps are not the same as restless legs syndrome. Both happen at night, but restless legs syndrome causes discomfort and the urge to move instead of painful muscle cramps. As much as they may hurt, nocturnal leg cramps are harmless.

Nocturnal Leg Cramp Causes and Risk Factors

Medical doctors, neurologists, and physiologists do not know the exact cause of nocturnal leg cramps. But, it could occur because your nerves send the wrong signals to the muscles. For example, your brain might mistakenly tell your leg to move while you dream, which confuses the calf muscles and causes them to contract.

You are more likely to have a leg cramp if you:

- Are 50 or older
- Do not drink enough water
- Sit too long without moving
- Stand too long on hard surfaces
- Work your muscles too much

Other health conditions may also raise your chances of leg cramps, including:

- Alcohol abuse
- ALS (amyotrophic lateral sclerosis/Lou Gehrig's disease)
- Blood flow problems
- Cirrhosis of the liver
- Congestive heart failure
- Diabetes

- Flat feet
- Hormone disorders, such as hypothyroidism
- Hypokalemia
- Kidney failure
- Low blood sugar
- Nerve damage
- Neurological disorders like Parkinson's disease
- Osteoarthritis
- Peripheral artery disease
- Peripheral neuropathy
- Pregnancy
- Too much or not enough of particular elements in the body, such as calcium, potassium, and magnesium

Some medications can cause leg cramps. These include:

- Albuterol/Ipratropium (Combivent®).
- Celecoxib (Celebrex®).
- Clonazepam (Klonopin®).
- Conjugated estrogens.
- Diuretics.
- Fluoxetine (Prozac®).
- Gabapentin (Neurontin®).
- Naproxen (Naprosyn®).
- Pregabalin (Lyrica®)
- Sertraline (Zoloft®).
- Statins.
- Zolpidem (Ambien®).

Leg cramps occur for no apparent reason. These are known as **idiopathic cramps**. Potential causes of these leg cramps include:

- Involuntary nerve discharges.
- Part of your leg muscle is not getting enough blood.

- Stress.
- Too much high-intensity exercise.

Nocturnal Leg Cramp Diagnosis

If you have severe leg cramps, talk to your doctor to be sure another problem is not causing them. They will ask about your medical history, symptoms and perform a physical exam to look for possible causes. You may require blood tests if your doctor suspects a hidden problem.

Treating Nocturnal Leg Cramps

The next time a nocturnal cramp happens, consider the following:

- Stretch the muscle.
- Get out of bed and stand with your foot flat on the floor. Press down firmly.
- Massage the muscle.
- Flex your foot.
- Grab your toes and pull them toward you.
- Ice the cramp.
- Take a warm bath.

What Medicines Help With Leg Cramps?

No medications can prevent leg cramps 100% of the time. However, some prescription medications show evidence of preventing some leg cramps. Under the guidance of your health care provider, you might try the following:

- Carisoprodol (Soma®): A muscle relaxant.
- Diltiazem (Cartia XT®): A calcium-channel blocker.
- Gabapentin (neurontin): Anticonvulsant and nerve pain medication.
- Magnesium.
- Orphenadrine (Norflex®): Treats muscle spasms and relieves pain and stiffness in muscles.
- Verapamil: A calcium-channel blocker.
- Vitamin B complex.

Can Vitamins Help With Leg Cramps?
No vitamin can help with a leg cramp 100% of the time, but some experts recommend taking vitamin B12 complex or magnesium.

CHAPTER 2
CAUSES and RISK FACTORS

THE PROBLEM

Most of the time, no apparent reason for nocturnal leg cramps can be readily detected. Nocturnal leg cramps are likely related to muscle fatigue and nerve problems. As one ages, the chance of getting nocturnal leg cramps increases. Pregnant women are also more likely to have nocturnal leg cramps than the general population.

The following should be noted:

- Multiple conditions, such as kidney failure and diabetic nerve damage, can cause nocturnal leg cramps. But, if you have one of these conditions, you are most likely aware of it and have symptoms other than nocturnal leg cramps.

- Although not proven scientifically, people taking certain medications, such as diuretics, are likelier to have nocturnal leg cramps.

- Restless Legs Syndrome (RLS) might be mistaken for nocturnal leg cramps, but it is a different condition.

In addition to the above, other conditions may be associated with nocturnal leg cramps, such as:

Structural Disorders:

Peripheral artery disease - is the reduction of arteries resulting in reduced blood flow, usually to the legs.

Spinal stenosis - is when the spinal column narrows and compresses the spinal cord.

Circulatory Disorders:

Atherosclerosis - blocks blood flow in the arteries. This pain, called claudication, is generally felt when exercising or walking and is relieved through resting.

Blood clot (deep vein thrombosis) - from long-term bed rest.

Infection of the bone (osteomyelitis) - soft tissue cellulitis.

Inflammation - of the leg joints caused by arthritis or gout.

Nerve damage - is familiar to people with diabetes, smokers, and alcoholics.

Varicose veins - a disorder in which the veins enlarge due to malfunctioning of their valves, causing improper blood flow and pooling.

Metabolic Problems:

Acute kidney failure - occurs when kidneys lose their ability to filter waste from the blood system.

Addison's disease - is a long-term endocrine disorder resulting from insufficient amounts of hormones released by the adrenal glands.

Anemia - a state in which the hemoglobin in blood is below the referenced range.

Chronic kidney disease - a condition measured by a gradual loss of kidney function.

Cirrhosis - a degenerative disorder of the liver resulting in scarring and liver failure.

Hyperthyroidism - an overactive thyroid.

Type 1 diabetes - a chronic condition where the pancreas produces little or no insulin.

Type 2 diabetes - a result of insufficient production of insulin, causing high blood sugar.

Medications and Procedures:

Blood pressure drugs - diuretics are some of the most used medications for treating high blood pressure. They help the kidneys eliminate excess water and sodium, thereby reducing the volume of blood that needs to pass through blood vessels (which lowers blood pressure).

Cholesterol-lowering drugs - statins are the first drug doctors prescribe to lower LDL.

Dialysis - the entire process of removing excess water, solutes, and toxins from the blood in individuals whose kidneys cannot perform these functions naturally.

Diuretics - a substance that promotes diuresis, an increase in urine production.

Oral contraceptives - birth-control pills (used to prevent pregnancy).

Statins - are a class of drugs that lowers cholesterol levels in the blood by reducing cholesterol production by the liver.

Other Conditions:

Dehydration - or small amounts of potassium, sodium, calcium, or magnesium in the blood.

Diarrhea - feces are discharged from the bowels frequently and in a liquid form. This condition may be caused by stress, anxiety, and antibiotics.

Muscle fatigue or strain - from overuse, too much exercise, or keeping a muscle in a position for a long time.

Strain - caused by a torn or overstretched muscle.

Stress fracture - or a hairline crack in the bone.

Nerve damage - from cancer treatments.

Osteoarthritis - a disease that causes the breakdown of joints.

Tendinitis - or an inflamed tendon.

Shin splints - the pain at the front of the leg from overuse.

Parkinson's disease - a continuing nervous system disorder that affects movement.

Pregnancy - leg cramps are common in the second and third trimesters.

Less Common Causes Can Include:

Cancerous bone tumors (osteosarcoma, Ewing sarcoma).

Legg-Calve-Perthes disease (insufficient blood flow to the hip that may stop or slow average leg growth).

Noncancerous (benign) tumors or cysts of the femur or tibia (osteoid osteoma).

Sciatic nerve pain caused by a slipped disk (radiating pain down the leg).

Slipped capital femoral epiphysis is commonly found in boys and overweight children ages 11 through 15.

Leg Cramps at Night

Low magnesium is the primary cause of muscle cramps everywhere in the body (including leg and foot cramps). The problem is that only 80% of Americans have enough magnesium within their body. **Magnesium is a necessary nutrient vital for health!**

Fixing a Magnesium Deficiency to Halt Cramps

To remedy a magnesium deficiency is FAST, EASY, SAFE, and POWERFUL. This vital mineral could:

- Dampen inflammation in the muscles and the entire body.

- Increases serotonin and melatonin, which helps you relax and fall asleep.

- It boosts the absorption of potassium, which is critical for proper muscle functioning.

- It relaxes blood vessels and decreases blood pressure, which restores healthy circulation.

- It relaxes the muscles by blocking the effect of calcium, which tightens them. With age, excess calcium collects in the muscles, causing cramps.

- Reduces pain by blocking pain receptors in the brain and nervous system.

NOTE	Magnesium is a necessary nutrient, not a medication. Health officials are saying that many people are walking around with magnesium levels that, while "sufficient," might be somewhat too low for optimal performance.

What is Magnesium?

It is a mineral that is essential to the human body's functions. Its primary role in the body is to act as a cofactor that enables the activation of critical biological enzymes. More than 300 enzymes require magnesium to function, including the biological pathways responsible for energy production, synthesis of DNA and RNA, blood sugar control, nerve and muscle cell function, immunity, hormone production, and many other essential processes.

Although magnesium is found naturally in certain foods, eating the recommended daily amount can be challenging, and that is why most people boost their diet with a magnesium supplement.

Why Magnesium is Crucial for Health

Adenosine triphosphate (ATP) is the principal energy molecule in the human body. It is a coenzyme that transports chemical energy within cells and is responsible for proper metabolism.

Magnesium is required to bond with phosphates to protect ATP molecules from degrading at high pH levels.

Additionally:

Magnesium is crucial for protein synthesis. Without it, ribozymes cannot locate the proper location and cannot synthesize new proteins. The proteins created by this process control the activities and growth of cells. Magnesium is also needed to produce DNA and RNA molecules.

Magnesium (1.5-2.5 mEq/L) is a crucial electrolyte. Along with sodium (136-145 mEq/L), potassium (5-5.3 mEq/L), chloride (97-107 mEq/L), and calcium (5-5.5 mEq/L), magnesium is an electrolyte found in mEq/L the body. As a positively charged ion, magnesium plays a significant role in maintaining homeostasis in the body and helps to balance the electrolyte levels in cells. *The figures in brackets are normal ranges.*

Magnesium helps to regulate other nutrient levels in the body. It is especially crucial for controlling the movement of calcium into the skeletal and smooth muscle cells, nerve cells, heart pacemaker cells, and other tissues. Although calcium is vital to the human body, too much can lead to anxiety, depression, insomnia, heart palpitations, asthma, cramps, muscle spasms, and chronic headaches. A magnesium deficiency means excess calcium will adversely affect cells throughout the body.

Besides regulating calcium movement, magnesium is necessary for ensuring that vitamin D, copper, zinc, sodium, and potassium are correctly used in various biological processes.

NOTE	Magnesium is necessary for the healthy functioning of many parts of the body. It can prevent kidney stones, fibromyalgia, depression, deafness, diabetes, insulin resistance, osteoporosis, migraines, preeclampsia and eclampsia, premenstrual syndrome, restless leg syndrome, colorectal cancer, and blood clots. It helps regulate cholesterol levels and has laxative properties.

Internal Processing of Magnesium

Magnesium is a positively charged ion, otherwise known as a cation. Therefore, it must be bonded with another compound before being consumed in either supplement or dietary form. Magnesium is typically connected with mixtures such as oxide, citrate, or chloride to help deliver it to the intestines when taken as a supplement. Once processed in the intestines, magnesium and the compound to which it is bonded will dissociate, leaving the magnesium free to perform its many roles. The kidneys play a crucial role in conserving and excreting magnesium, depending on the level in the body.

NOTE	50 to 60% of all magnesium in the human body is stored in the bones. Less than 1% is found in blood and blood serum, and the balance is in the body's soft tissues.

What Does a Magnesium Deficiency Do?
With a magnesium deficiency, the body cannot function properly, and you could develop muscle weakness, depression, high blood pressure, and even heart disease.

This mineral is vital for **'regulation'** and helps:

- The brain communicates with the body.
- The heart maintains a healthy beat.
- Muscles regulate their contractions.
- Blood pressure stays low.

NOTE	Every muscle in the body depends on magnesium to keep and continue working correctly.

Magnesium Deficiency Signs and Symptoms
Magnesium deficiency looks like many other conditions since magnesium involves many body processes. Trying to pinpoint magnesium deficiency as the source of specific troubles, especially when the mineral is involved in so many seemingly unrelated functions in the body, is difficult.

The following are the most common signs of low magnesium:

- Aches and pains
- ADHD
- Anxiety
- Arrhythmias
- Brain fog
- Constipation
- Depression

- Digestive trouble
- Fatigue
- Heart irregularities, palpitations, or flutters
- Irregular sleep patterns and insomnia
- Lack of appetite
- Memory problems
- Migraines
- Mood problems
- Muscle cramps
- Muscle cramps and spasms
- Nightly leg cramps, especially during pregnancy
- PMS
- Restless leg syndrome
- Twitching eyelids, lips, or skeletal muscle

NOTE	Some of the above symptoms can have a root cause other than a magnesium deficiency. Conditions can be severe and require medical attention. Review all your concerns with your doctor.

Why Are So Many People Magnesium Deficient?

It is estimated that over 80% of people are magnesium deficient. But why so many? You do not get as much magnesium in your diet as your predecessors. Magnesium deficiency is a modern phenomenon primarily caused by industrial farming and food processing techniques that depleted ground soil and crops of their former magnesium content. The typical American diet provides only half of the Recommended

Daily Allowance (RDA) of magnesium. Consequently, most Americans are, to some extent, deficient in magnesium. Older adults are more deficient in magnesium because their intestines absorb less, and their kidneys excrete more than younger adults.

Other causes include:
Reduced nutrient density in modern diets (reliance on pre-packaged foods). And increased magnesium excretion (reduced absorption) triggered by stress, caffeine, sugar intake, and some pharmaceuticals.

The Magnesium RBC Test

The magnesium RBC test measures the amount of magnesium stored in your **'red blood cells.'** It indicates how much magnesium your body reserves in your bones and soft tissues.

The Optimal Magnesium Range

If your numbers are below 6.0 mg/dl, you will want to supplement, and if your lab results are reported in mmol/L, multiply that number by 2.43 to get mg/dl and see how close you are to 6.0, a **functional level.**

Most labs report a normal range, which tells you more about the levels of everyone else's magnesium than it tells you about the amount your body needs to work correctly.

CHAPTER 3
SOURCING MAGNESIUM

Recommended Daily Allowance For Magnesium

The following table exhibits the recommended daily allowance (RDA) or adequate intake for men and women in the United States.

AGE	MALE	FEMALE	PREGNANCY	LACTATION
Birth to 6 mo.	30 mg. *	30 mg. *		
7-12 mo.	75 mg.	75 mg.		
1-3 years	80 mg.	80 mg.		
4–8 years	130 mg.	80 mg.		
9–13 years	240 mg.	80 mg.		
14–18 years	410 mg.	80 mg.	400 mg	360 mg
19–30 years	400 mg.	80 mg.	350 mg	310 mg
31–50 years	420 mg	320 mg	360 mg	320 mg
51+ years	420 mg	320 mg		

*Adequate intake

Proper Dosage and Contraindications

There are different recommendations for how much magnesium people should ingest each day, depending on age, gender, and other factors. The Food and Nutrition Board at the Institute of Medicine of the National Academies defined the Recommended Dietary Allowance (RDA). The Mayo Clinic has similar yet slightly lower recommendations and other healthcare professionals recommend more magnesium for adults. You should not administer magnesium supplements to a child without a doctor's **permission.**

NOTE	When you supplement, research shows that the body absorbs magnesium best when taken in doses of 100 to 125 mg at a time. If more is taken, the body is much less efficient at absorbing it due to intestinal permeability limits, so it will just pass through the body. Also, the body needs an adequate level of vitamin B6 to process magnesium correctly.

NATURAL FORMS OF MAGNESIUM

Dark, leafy vegetables such as spinach, swiss chard, and kale are the best dietary sources of magnesium, followed by nuts and seeds. Certain fruits, peas, beans, soy products, and whole grains contain magnesium, as do wheat bran, oatmeal, chocolate, meat, seafood, and milk.

Vegetables

VEGETABLE	SERVING	MAGNESIUM	
Spinach	3.5 oz., 100g.	80 mg.	
Swiss Chard	3.5 oz., 100g.	80 mg.	
Kale	3.5 oz., 100g.	50 mg.	
Romaine Lettuce	3.5 oz., 100g.	15 mg.	

Nuts and Seeds

NUT / SEED	SERVING	MAGNESIUM	
Almonds	1.0 oz., 28g.	78 mg.	
Pumpkin Seeds	1.0 oz., 28g.	73 mg.	
Walnuts	1.0 oz., 28g.	56 mg.	
Peanuts	1.0 oz., 28g.	50 mg.	
Hazelnuts	1.0 oz., 28g.	49 mg.	
Sunflower Seeds	1.0 oz., 28g.	33 mg.	

OTHER FORMS OF MAGNESIUM

Magnesium is Rich for Mood and Memory

Dark chocolate has 64 mg of magnesium in a 1-ounce (28-gram) serving. It is high in iron and copper and contains prebiotic fiber that feeds healthy gut bacteria. Dark chocolate contains magnesium and tryptophan and offers a dual approach to enhancing mood and mental clarity. Tryptophan is the precursor to serotonin, the brain chemical that makes you feel happy, focused, and calm.

Vegetable - Magnesium Rich and Fiber

These vegetables will help you go more regularly:

- Artichokes
- Asparagus
- Avocados
- Broccoli
- Cabbage
- Legumes
- Spinach (lightly steam it first to reduce the lectin content)

Other Foods That Are Magnesium Rich and Fiber

The following is a two-for: plenty of magnesium and other healthy goodies.

Fatty fish - many fish are high in magnesium and rich in potassium, selenium, B vitamins, and other nutrients. These fish include salmon, mackerel, and halibut.

Bananas - are among the most popular fruits in the world and are rich in magnesium. Well-known for their high potassium content, bananas provide vitamin C, B6, manganese, and fiber.

SUPPLEMENTS

Magnesium Found in Supplements

There are several magnesium forms, and each has its pros and cons:

Magnesium oxide and hydroxide - supplement companies love this because it is cheap. Unfortunately, it is poorly absorbed (only 8%) and is highly laxative. It is what you find in most common multivitamins. It is also the active ingredient in **Milk of Magnesia.**

Magnesium citrate - well absorbed and highly laxative. It is the main ingredient in many laxatives. For those that have had a colonoscopy, this is what they provided to **'clean you out.'**

Magnesium sulfate - also known as **Epsom Salt,** is a good laxative.

Magnesium glycinate - is magnesium bound to the amino acid glycine. This form is unrealistic because magnesium tells your neurons to slow down, and glycine tells them to speed up. So, do magnesium and glycine cancel each other out?

Magnesium chelate or glutamate - both are the same thing. These products are low quality because they have large amounts of **'unbound magnesium.'** This form of magnesium causes laxative effects.

Magnesium chloride - turns into a liquid when exposed to air, which makes it difficult to deliver via capsule. It is not found in food naturally.

Magnesium taurinate - this is a magnesium bound to the amino acid Taurine. It has a side effect of causing extreme drowsiness, making it difficult to take during the day. It is also expensive.

Because magnesium is an ion, it is commercially available as an oral supplement only when combined with a carrier. It binds and carries it to the intestines, where it is broken down into elemental magnesium and used throughout the body. Different carriers break apart at different rates, which affects the bioavailability of essential magnesium and how much can be absorbed by the body.

Magnesium supplements should always be taken with meals. Taking some magnesium supplements on an empty stomach could cause diarrhea.

Items to Avoid When Choosing Supplements
Vitamin D and Fillers - be wary of any supplement containing ergocalciferol (D2), cholecalciferol (D3), and artificial or unnecessary ingredients or fillers. They are useless and can cause uncomfortable and dangerous side effects.

Pay attention to the dosage. You will see supplements with as little as 20 mg of magnesium, which is ineffective. Although, it is not as simple as **'more is better.'** i.e., taking too much synthetic, low-quality D3 can harm your health.

Very High Dosages - many nutrients taken in large quantities can cause health complications and unnecessary strain on your liver and other organs.

Unknown Manufacturers - the product's label should be understandable, and you should be able to verify any claims made by the company before you buy their supplement. Select well-known manufacturers only.

Vitamins and Supplements Additives?

Manufacturers put additives into vitamin and supplement tablets and capsules as a processing aid. The following are of no benefit to your body.

Anti-caking agents - to stop the ingredients from clogging up machines.

Binders - are used to stick ingredients together in a tablet.

Bulking agents - to top off the content of the pills or capsules.

Carriers - to maintain a powder consistency.

Coatings - to make swallowing easy.

Colors - to look more appealing to the consumer.

Emulsifiers - to bind water to fats.

Fillers - add to the volume of tablets and capsules.

Flavors - to alter the taste, even in tablets that are swallowed whole.

Preservatives - to save ingredients from spoiling.

Sweeteners - to make the flavor more palatable.

Caution, Potentially Harmful Additives

Choose additive-free products. The following additives may be potentially harmful:

Magnesium stearate and stearic acid are used in 90% of nutritional supplements to speed manufacturing and keep costs down. It can be derived from animals or vegetables, has no nutritional benefit, and could cause harm.

Dicalcium phosphate is a cheap and inorganic form of calcium that helps bulk out tablets. It is not well absorbed and used by the body.

Gelatin is an animal protein that is not vegan-friendly and is likely to be sourced from low-quality, factory-farmed animals fed GMO grain.

Lactose is sugar from milk, likely sourced from cows treated with medications and fed grains. It is also a common allergen.

Sodium selenite and selenite are toxic, inorganic chemical sources of selenium.

Titanium dioxide is a colorant used for making tablets and capsules bright white. It is not an ingredient found in any natural food.

NOTE	Most vitamins and minerals contain synthetic laboratory-produced materials. Because the materials are artificially made (not from natural food), your body is not guaranteed to recognize or use them.

Be Safe - Choose Chemical-Free Supplements

- Select natural products from food sources.
- Read the labels and look up any questionable ingredients.
- Check for Good Manufacturing Practices (GMP) certification and vigorous quality control.

Magnesium and Prescribed Drugs

Magnesium has been known to interfere with more than 30 prescribed drugs. For optimal effectiveness, avoid combining a magnesium supplement with the following medications: aminoglycosides, antibiotics (ciprofloxacin, moxifloxacin, tetracycline, doxycycline, minocycline), blood pressure medications, calcium channel blockers (amlodipine, diltiazem, felodipine, verapamil), diabetes medications, digoxin, diuretics, fluoroquinolones, hormone replacement therapy, labetalol, levomethadyl, levothyroxine, penicillamine, tiludronate and alendronate, amphotericin B, corticosteroids, antacids, and insulin. Seek advice from a health care professional before taking magnesium simultaneously with any of these medications.

Dosing magnesium is difficult and uncommon because the kidneys excrete excess amounts into the urine. However, there is a limit to how much the kidneys can do. As soon as this limit is reached, there can be negative consequences. Diarrhea is the most common side effect of excessive magnesium intake, and it can be accompanied by nausea and abdominal cramping as the body excretes excessive magnesium.

Severe magnesium overdose can result in additional problems such as kidney failure, severely lowered blood pressure and heart problems. But, to overdose, one must consume an exorbitantly large amount of magnesium.

CHAPTER 4
HOME CARE and HEALTHCARE

Home Care

If you suffer from leg pain caused by cramps or overuse, try these steps first:

- Rest as much as possible.

- Elevate your leg.

- Apply ice for up to 15 minutes. Do this four times daily, more often for the first few days.

- Gently stretch and massage cramping muscles.

- Take over-the-counter pain medicines like acetaminophen or ibuprofen.

- Other home care will depend on the cause of your leg pain.

Activities that might help relieve night leg cramps include:

- Flexing your foot up toward your head.

- Massaging the cramped muscle with your hands or with ice.

- Walking or jiggling the leg.

- Take a hot shower or warm bath.

When Should I See My Health Care Provider?

See your health care provider if your leg cramps are unbearably painful, frequent, or last long. Additionally, consult your provider immediately if you have any of the following symptoms in addition to the leg cramps:

- Changes in the skin of your leg.
- Muscle cramps in other parts of your body.
- Significant pain.
- Swelling or numbness in your leg.
- The leg cramps stop you from getting enough sleep.
- The leg is black and blue.
- The leg is cold and pale.
- The painful leg is swollen or red.
- Waking up over and over again with leg cramps.
- You are taking medicines that may be causing leg pain. DO NOT stop taking or changing your medication without talking to your provider.
- You have a fever.
- You have fluid abnormalities or electrolyte imbalances.

Questions to Ask Your Health Care Provider

You might want to ask your provider the following:

- Can you tell me the best exercises that I can do to stretch my muscles?

- Can you show me the best massage techniques to help my leg cramps?

- Would you suggest I see a physical therapist, sleep specialist, massage therapist, or other specialist?

- Do you believe that my leg cramping is a symptom of an underlying condition?

- How can I help my child when they have a leg cramp?

- How often should I come back to visit you about my leg cramps?

- Is it safe for me to take medication for my leg cramps? Which medicines should I take?

- Should I watch for symptoms other than leg cramps that could indicate a more serious condition?

When Should I Go To The ER?

Go to the emergency room if a leg cramp lasts longer than 10 minutes or becomes unbearably painful. Also, go if a leg cramp happens after you touch a substance that could be poisonous or infectious. For example, if you have a cut on your skin that touches dirt, you could get a bacterial infection like tetanus. Exposure to mercury, lead, or other toxic substances should also be a reason to go to the emergency department.

APPENDIX - A

GLOSSARY

WORD	MEANING
Cofactor	A substance whose presence is essential for the activity of an enzyme.
DNA	Deoxyribonucleic acid - the genetic material in humans and almost all other organisms.
Electrolyte	An electrolyte is a medium containing ions that are electrically conducted through the movement of those ions but not conducting electrons. This includes most soluble salts, acids, and bases dissolved in a polar solvent like water. The substance dissolves into cations and anions, which disperse uniformly throughout the solvent.
LDL Cholesterol	Often called bad cholesterol because it could build up in the walls of arteries and form plaque, putting you at risk for a cardiovascular issue such as a heart attack or stroke.
Milliequivalents per liter (mEq/L)	Note: some medical tests report milliequivalents per liter (mEq/L) results. An equivalent is the amount of a substance that will react with a certain number of hydrogen ions. A milliequivalent is one-thousandth of an equivalent. A liter is a fluid volume measurement of slightly more than a quart.
Ph	A scale is used to specify how acidic or basic a water-based solution is. Acidic solutions have a lower pH, while essential solutions have a higher ph. At room temperature, **pure water is neither acidic nor basic and has a neutral pH 7.0.**

Restless Leg Syndrome (RLS)	RLS disorder causes an unpleasant feeling in the legs that improves somewhat with moving them. The feeling is described as aching, tingling, or crawling. RLS often occurs at rest, making it hard to sleep. Due to a disturbance in sleep, people with RLS may have daytime sleepiness, low energy, irritability, and a depressed mood. **RLS** is often confused with **Night Leg Cramps,** but it is a different condition.
RNA	Ribonucleic acid is a polymeric molecule implicated in various biological roles in the coding, decoding, regulating, and expressing genes.

VITAMINS and MINERALS

ITEM	DESCRIPTION
VITAMINS	
A	A group of unsaturated nutritional organic compounds includes retinol, retinal, retinoic acid, and several provitamins A carotenoids. Vitamin A has multiple functions - it is essential for growth and development, the maintenance of the immune system, and good vision. The eye's retina needs it as a retinal, combined with protein opsin, to form rhodopsin, the light-absorbing molecule required for both low-light and color vision. Vitamin A functions differently from retinoic acid, an essential hormone-like growth factor for epithelial and other cells.
B	Any of a group of substances (the vitamin B complex) that are essential for working certain enzymes in the body and, although not chemically related, are usually found together in the same foods. They include vitamins - B1, B2, B6, and B12.
B1	Thiamine - a vitamin found in foods and produced as a dietary supplement and medication. Food sources of thiamine include whole grains, legumes, and some meats and fish.
B2	Riboflavin - is a vitamin found in food and used as a dietary supplement. Food sources include eggs, green vegetables, milk, other dairy products, meat, mushrooms, and almonds.
B3	Niacin - also called nicotinic acid. It occurs naturally in plants and animals.
B6	Pyridoxine - is a group of chemically similar compounds that can be interconverted in biological systems. It is an essential nutrient. In its active form, pyridoxal phosphate is a coenzyme in some 100 enzyme reactions in amino acid, glucose, and lipid metabolism.
B12	Cyanocobalamin - is a water-soluble vitamin that

	plays an essential role in red blood cell formation, cell metabolism, nerve function, and the production of DNA. Food sources include poultry, meat, fish, and dairy products. A deficiency is rare because the body can store several years' worth of B-12. However, following a vegetarian or vegan diet might lead to deficiency because plant foods do not contain vitamin B-12. Older adults and people with digestive tract conditions that affect nutrient absorption are susceptible to vitamin B-12 deficiency. Untreated, a deficiency can lead to anemia, fatigue, muscle weakness, intestinal problems, nerve damage, and mood disturbances.
C	Ascorbic acid and L-ascorbic acid - are vitamins found in various foods. It is used to prevent and treat scurvy. This vitamin is an essential nutrient involved in tissue repair and the enzymatic production of certain neurotransmitters. It is required for the functioning of several enzymes and is necessary for immune system function. It also functions as an antioxidant.
D2	Ergocalciferol - also known as calciferol, is a type of vitamin D found in food and used as a dietary supplement. As a supplement, it is used to prevent and treat vitamin D deficiency.
D3	Cholecalciferol - is used as a dietary supplement by people who do not get enough vitamin D to maintain adequate health.
E	A vitamin is found in many foods, including vegetable oils, cereals, meat, poultry, eggs, fruits, vegetables, and wheat germ oil.

MINERALS	
Copper	Copper is a mineral found in many foods, especially organ meats, seafood, nuts, seeds, wheat bran cereals, grain products, and cocoa products. The body stores copper mainly in the bones and muscles. The liver regulates the amount of copper in the blood. There is no evidence that people who eat a regular diet need a copper supplement.
Potassium	A mineral that is crucial for life. It is necessary for the heart, kidneys, and other organs to work normally. Most people that eat a healthy diet should get enough potassium naturally. Low potassium is associated with a risk of high blood pressure, heart disease, stroke, arthritis, cancer, digestive disorders, and infertility.
Sodium	Table salt is a combination of two minerals, sodium and chloride. The body needs some sodium to work properly. It helps with the function of nerves, muscles and helps maintain the right balance of fluids in your body. The kidneys control how much sodium is in your body. If you have too much and your kidneys cannot eliminate it, sodium builds up in your blood, leading to high blood pressure.
Zinc	An essential nutrient that plays many roles in the body. The body does not produce zinc, which must be obtained through food or supplements. Zinc is necessary for numerous processes in the body.

ABOUT SUPPLEMENTS

Dietary supplements may be beneficial at any age but can have unwanted side effects, such as unsafe prescription drug interactions. They could also not work at all. Understanding your supplements and why you are taking them is essential. Consult your doctor if you are thinking about a supplement.

What Is a Dietary Supplement?
Dietary supplements are substances you could use to add nutrients to your diet or reduce your risk of health-related issues. Supplements are available in pills, capsules, powders, gel capsules, tablets, extracts, and liquids. They may contain vitamins, minerals, fiber, amino acids, herbs or other plants, or enzymes. A prescription is not needed to buy dietary supplements.

Should I Take a Dietary Supplement?
Eating healthy foods is the best way to obtain the nutrients you need. Still, some people may not get enough vitamins and minerals from their daily diet. When that is the case, their doctors may recommend a dietary supplement to supply the missing nutrients.

If you are thinking about using dietary supplements:

Tell your doctor - before you take a dietary supplement to help treat any health condition, check with your doctor. Do not take a supplement to diagnose or treat any medical condition without first checking with your doctor.

Learn - learn as much as possible about any dietary supplement you might take. Talk with your doctor, pharmacist, or registered dietitian. A supplement that worked for someone else may not work for you. If you read fact sheets or websites, be aware of the source of information. *Could the writer or group profit from selling a particular supplement*

Remember - because something is said to be **"natural"** does not mean it is safe or suitable for you. It could have side effects or make the medicine your doctor prescribed for you weaker or stronger. It might also be harmful if you have certain medical conditions.

Buy wisely - choose brands your doctor, dietitian, or pharmacist recommends. Do not buy dietary supplements with ingredients you do not need. Do not assume more is better. Taking too many supplements or having a very high nutrient concentration can be harmful. You can waste money on unneeded supplements.

Check the science - to ensure that any claim in connection with a dietary supplement is based on scientific evidence. Look for the **United States Pharmacopeia (USP)** verified mark. USP verifies the identity, quality, strength, and purity of supplements. Information on certain dietary supplements is available at **MedlinePlus,** but it is important to note that most listed supplements have limited evidence of any benefit. If something sounds too good to be true, it probably is.

Are Dietary Supplements Safe?

The **U.S. Food and Drug Administration (FDA)** checks prescription medicines, such as antibiotics or blood pressure drugs, to ensure they are safe and do what they promise. The same is true for over-the-counter medications such as pain and cold medicines.

The FDA does not have authority over dietary supplements. They do not have to be approved by the agency for safety or efficacy before being sold to the public.

The federal government does not test what is in dietary supplements, and the companies are not required to share information about the safety of these products with the FDA before they sell them. That is why just because the dietary supplement is on a store shelf does not mean it is safe, does what the label says it will, or contains what it states. If the FDA receives reports of possible problems with a supplement, it will issue warnings about the product. The FDA may also take supplements found to be unsafe off the market.

The Federal Trade Commission investigates reports of ads that may misrepresent what dietary supplements do. Private organizations, such as the **U.S. Pharmacopeia, NSF International, ConsumerLab.com,** and the **Natural Products Association,** have their own **"seals of approval"** for dietary supplements. To earn the seal, the products must be made by following reasonable production processes, must contain what is listed on the label, and must not have unsafe levels of ingredients that do not belong there, such as lead.

Whether you take dietary supplements or not, following a healthy lifestyle is still important. Try a nutritious diet, being physically active, keeping your mind busy, not smoking, and seeing your doctor regularly.

WHAT IS THE DIFFERENCE BETWEEN

Disease, Disorder, Condition, and Syndrome

A disease is a pathophysiological response to internal or external factors. A disease is a medical condition with a known and understood reason behind it. The disease is the highest level of conceptual understanding of medical issues. It means the medical community knows all the underlying causes in the case of a disease.

A disorder is a disruption to regular bodily structure and function. A disorder is a disruption in the normal functioning of the mind or body due to disease, genetic factors, or trauma. Arrhythmia or irregular heartbeat, for example, is a disruption in the normal functioning of the heart due to cardiovascular diseases. It is not a disease in itself. Disorders may be classified into the following areas:

- Behavioral
- Emotional
- Genetic
- Mental
- Physical
- Structural

A condition is an abnormal state of health that interferes with normal feelings of well-being. The condition is an abnormal physical or mental health state that interferes with usual activities or the sense of well-being.

A syndrome is a collection of signs and symptoms associated with a specific health-related cause. The syndrome is a set or collection of identifying signs and symptoms that characterize certain diseases or disorders. A syndrome (a Greek word meaning 'run together') may produce symptoms without an identifiable cause.

Health care vs. Healthcare
The difference between the word health care (two words) refers to provider actions. Healthcare (one word) is the system. Health care is the specific things people do: see a patient or prescribe medication. Healthcare is an industry, the system by which people get the necessary health care.

Doctor vs. Physician
The primary distinction between doctors and physicians is that a doctor is any person who has earned a doctoral degree in any field. In contrast, physicians have completed medical school and residency training to provide health management and health care. They are medical doctors.

Patient vs. Person
A patient is a sick individual, especially when waiting or under the care and treatment of a physician or surgeon, and a person is a human considered an individual.

Therapy vs. Treatment
The difference between therapy and treatment is that the word therapy is used in the sense of rehabilitation. On the other hand, the word treatment is used in the sense of cure. It is the main difference between the two words.

Type vs. Form

A simple way to distinguish between the two is to use type when classifying or grouping something while using form when discussing the structure and make of something.

APPENDIX - B

ACKNOWLEDGMENT

We acknowledge the following ARTICLES, which provided information for the content of this publication. Additionally, the indicated ORGANIZATIONS are authoritative in the fields of the content presented in this publication.

REFERENCED ARTICLES

AACM Staff. (2021). What are sleep leg cramps? American Academy of Sleep Medicine, https://sleepeducation.org/sleep-disorders/sleep-leg-cramps/

CDC Staff. (2022) Sleep and sleep Disorders - Basics About Sleep. CDC, https://www.cdc.gov/sleep/about_sleep/index.html

Mayo Clinic Staff. (2019). Sleep Disorders – Overview. Mayo Clinic, https://www.mayoclinic.org/diseases-conditions/sleep-disorders/symptoms-causes/syc-20354018

McMillen, M. (2022) Nocturnal Leg Cramps. WebMD, https://www.webmd.com/sleep-disorders/leg-cramps

Leg Cramps at Night: Causes, Treatment, Prevention, and Seeking Help https://www.healthline.com/health/leg-cramps-at-night

Vandergriendt, C. (2023). What's Causing Your Leg Cramps at Night? Treatment and Prevention Tips. Healthline, https://www.healthline.com/health/leg-cramps-at-night

ORGANIZATIONS

American Academy of Sleep Medicine (AASM)
2510 N. Frontage Road | Darien, IL 60561
630.737.9700
info@sleepeducation.org

Centers for Disease Control and Prevention
1600 Clifton Road | Atlanta, GA 30329-4027
800-232-4636 (800-CDC-INFO)
https://www.cdc.gov/sleep/index.html

Center for Food Safety and Applied Nutrition (CFSAN)
888-723-3366
https://www.fda.gov/about-fda/fda-organization/center-food-safety-and-applied-nutrition-cfsan

National Heart, Lung, and Blood Institute (NHLBI)
301-592-8573
nhlbiinfo@nhlbi.nih.gov
www.nhlbi.nih.gov

The Food and Nutrition Board (FNB) Institute of Medicine
500 Fifth Street, NW, Room K-739 | Washington, DC 20001
202-334-1732 (Voice)
202-334-2316 (FAX)

The U.S. Food and Drug Administration (FDA)
10903 New Hampshire Ave. | Silver Spring, MD 20993
1-888-INFO-FDA (1-888-463-6332)
https://www.usa.gov/federal-agencies/food-and-drug-administration

The Environmental Working Group (EWG)
1436 U Street NW, Suite 100 | Washington, DC 20009
(202) 667-6982
https://www.ewg.org/

ABOUT THE AUTHOR

Pierre Mouchette is a real estate investor, entrepreneur, and author of expository publications on **Real Estate Investing and Investment Knowledge, Environmental Knowledge, Life Knowledge, and Life-Health Knowledge.** All work produced involves critical-thinking skills, simplifying complex, technical information for consumers with nontechnical backgrounds, research, analysis, and input from industry experts and national organizations. Publications explain, inform, describe, and present concepts in simple, understandable language. Expository content is appropriately structured in **Books, Manuals, Guides, and How-to-Articles.**

For more information on Pierre, click here.
{https://www.synchronicity-investor.com/about-author.html}.

THE TEAM

We acknowledge the following individuals who read our unpublished manuscript before its final editing. These Team Members are within the target audience and have volunteered to read the manuscript and give honest feedback on its contents. The Team Members take our work from good but not ready for publication to being prepared for a final edit.

CREDITS	
Alpha Readers	Tomasa Mouchette
Beta Readers	

AFTERWORD

Thank You For Reading,

NOCTURNAL LEG CRAMPS
And Other Leg Muscle Pains

We hope you enjoyed this
Enviro | Life Knowledge Publication

Thank you again, valued reader,
And we hope to meet you again on another book.

Suggested Reading:

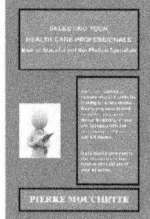

SELECTING YOUR HEALTH CARE PROFESSIONALS
Medical Specialists and Non-Medical Specialists
Organizations within the healthcare industry, such as doctor's offices and hospitals, almost always focus on guiding their practice by treating as many people as possible and as successfully as possible. It is an important priority that should remain. However, too often, this priority eclipses important business fundamentals like customer service, leaving unhappy patients who never return or eventually complain about the organization.

Choosing a doctor or hospital is essential, so you should give yourself as much information as possible. Not all physicians and health facilities are the same and do not provide the same level of care.

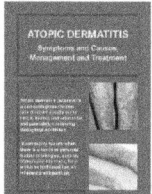

ATOPIC DERMATITIS
Symptoms and Causes, Management and Treatment
Atopic dermatitis (eczema) is a non-contagious chronic skin disorder usually occurring in infancy and childhood and potentially continuing throughout adulthood.

It commonly occurs when there is a family or personal history of allergies, such as asthma and hay fever, from which an individual has an inherent predisposition.

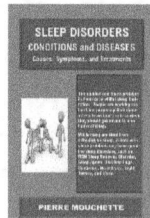

SLEEP DISORDERS – CONDITIONS and DISEASES
The number one sleep problem in America is willful sleep limitation. People are working too hard and purposely limit themselves to six hours or less when they should get seven to nine hours of sleep.

While many are tired from skimping on sleep, others with sleep problems may have genuine sleep disorders, such as REM Sleep Behavior Disorder, Sleep Apnea, Restless Legs Syndrome, Narcolepsy, Night Terrors, and More.

www.ingramcontent.com/pod-product-compliance
Lightning Source LLC
Chambersburg PA
CBHW062257290526
45794CB00006B/2583